A Short Profile of Antidiabetic Drugs

Profiles of Antidiabetics

A Short Profile of Antidiabetic Drugs

Profiles of Antidiabetics

Mohammed Abrar H. Malek

ELIVA PRESS

Published by Eliva Press
Email: info@elivapress.com
Website: www.elivapress.com

ISBN: 978-1-63648-319-1

Clinical Profile Analysis of Antidiabetic Drugs: An Overview

Mr. Mohammedabrar H. Malek

Department of Industrial Chemistry, V.P & R.P.T.P Science College

Affiliated to Sardar Patel University,

Vallabh Vidyanagar, Anand- Gujarat, India.

ABSTRACT

Over the late years, there has been quick development of various classes of antihyperglycemic drugs. These medications have various toxicological profiles in light of the fact that each has a one of a kind pharmacological system of activity and correspondingly. The antidiabetic drugs can possibly impact on patient ordinarily require for the clinical appraisal and treatment. So many varieties of anti-diabetic meds which are used for the curation of the diabetic mellitus type -II disease. This article is concise overview of the drugs which are used as oral hypoglycemic, administration and the other comparison and substitute medication to cure and to control the levels of sugar in human body and also gives information regarding their pharmacokinetics and pharmacodynamics properties.

KEYWORDS Anti-diabetics, 2nd Generation Sulphonylureas, Treatment for T2DM, Clinical Aspects.

1. INTRODUCTION

Extreme excretion of sweet urine' is the meaning of diabetes mellitus [1]. The disease diabetes mellitus is one of the diseases which is related to metabolic and generally define by the hypoglycemia [2] originated from pull out in the secretion of insulin. Association of chronic hyperglycemia of diabetes with long term in human body affect or damage, defunction and deficiency of numerous organs of human body especially in eyes, kidneys, nervous system, cardiac vessels and blood vessels. The reason behind the hyperglycemia take place in human body is because of the lesser secretion of insulin to the targeted cells. In hyperglycemia, the level of glucose in blood goes too high that which "overrun" in urine.

1.1 Causes of diabetes mellitus

The main causes of diabetes mellitus are as per hereditary deformities of beta-cell function [3]. Hereditary deformities in insulin activity. Illnesses of the exocrine pancreas. Endocrinopathies, i.e., changes in hormonal emission and, Drugs or synthetic incited.

1.2 Kinds of diabetes ellitus

Insulin reliant on or adolescent beginning diabetes mellitus (Type-I Diabetes mellitus) and Non-insulin reliant on or development beginning diabetes mellitus (Type-II Diabetes mellitus).

I) Type-I Diabetes Mellitus

Insulin dependent diabetes mellitus (IDDM), i.e., patients require occasional portions of insulin it can supervene at any age, ordinarily happens in kids, characterized by the stamped failure of the pancreas to discharge insulin in light of the fact that of immune system elimination of the β-cells. Kidney breaking down, nerve debilitation, cardiovascular malady also, retinal degeneration happens.

II) Type-II Diabetes Mellitus

Type-II diabetes is non-insulin dependent diabetes mellitus (NIDDM). It represents about 90%-92% of the analyzed cases of diabetes and influences 18% - 20 % of the populace more than 65 years old enough. Insulin receptors on insulin-responsive cells don't react ordinarily to insulin and are hence called as "insulin safe", in this manner expanding blood glucose level.

Here, we have discussed the drugs regarding the curation of the diabetes-II mellitus and their pharmacodynamics and pharmacokinetics profiles. The list of the drugs is mentioned in Table 1.

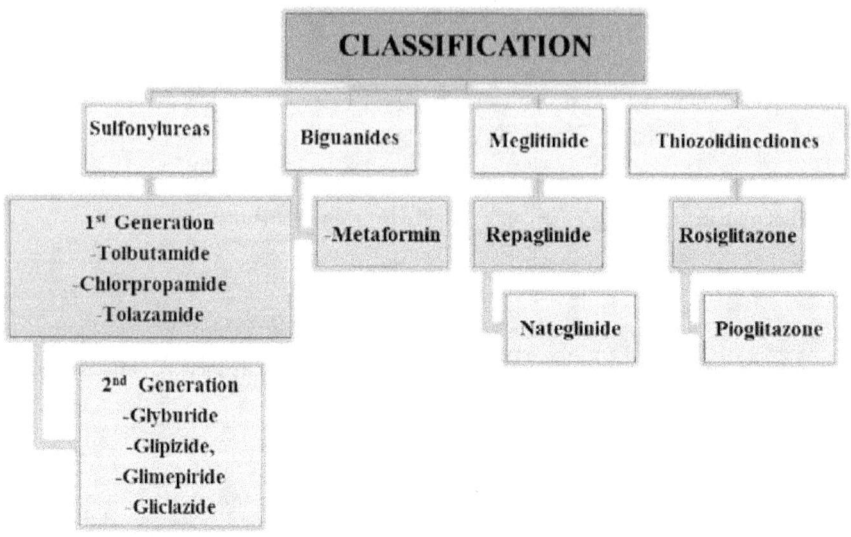

Figure 1. List of drugs used in curation of diabetes- II mellitus.

2. Profile Analysis Of Anti-Diabetic Drugs:

2.1 Gliclazide Drug Profile

The gliclazide an oral antihyperglycemic drug which is used and utilized for the curation of the disease called non- insulin dependent diabetes mellitus (NIDDM). It is classified under the sulfonylurea drug second class of insulin secretagogues, by which it acts as an invigorating- β cell of pancreas to deliver insulin [4].

2.2 Specifications of Gliclazide

2.2.1 IUPAC name

1-(4-methylbenzenesulfonyl)-3-{octahydrocyclopenta[c]pyrrol-2-yl} urea

2.2.2 Generic name

Diamicron, Glimicron

2.2.3 Molecular formula

$C_{15}H_{21}N_3O_3S$

2.2.4 Molecular weight

323.411   gm/mol

2.2.5 CAS registration number

21187-98-4

2.2.6 Structural formula

The structure of gliclazide is shown in Fig. 1.

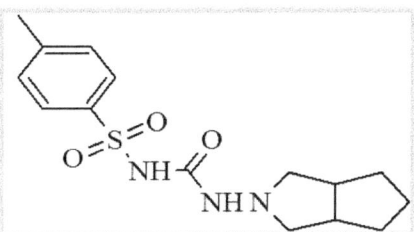

Fig. 2 Structure of gliclazide drug.

2.2.7 Physicochemical properties of gliclazide

2.2.7.1 Melting point

180- 182 °C

2.2.7.2 Appearance

A white or almost white powder

2.2.7.3 Solubility

The solubilization in some organic and inorganic solvents are shown and mentioned in Table 1.

Solvent Used	Solubility
Water & alcohol	Insoluble
Methylene chloride	Freely soluble
Acetone	Sparingly soluble
Ethanol (96%)	Slightly soluble

Table 1 Solubilization data of gliclazide.

2.2.7.4 pKa

14.13

2.2.7.5 Therapeutic categories

Gliclazide is under categorized to an Oral antidiabetic agent.

2.2.7.6 Boiling point

Not applicable

2.2.7.7 Mechanism of action

Gliclazide ties to the ß cell sulfonylurea receptor. This coupling thusly hinders the ATP susceptive potassium channels. The coupling brings about the conclusion of the channels and prompts a subsequent lessening in potassium efflux prompts depolarization of the ß-cells. This opens voltage-subordinate calcium directs in the ß-cell coming about in calmodulin enactment, which thus prompts exocytosis of insulin-containing secretory granules.

2.2.8 Clinical pharmacokinetics properties of gliclazide

2.2.8.1 Absorption

Quickly and all-around assimilated however may have wide between and intra-singular fluctuation. Pinnacle plasma focuses happen inside 4-6 hours of the oral organization.

2.2.8.2 Distribution

Gliclazide is circulated in the extracellular liquid, prompting to high concentrations in the internal organs of the human body (liver, kidneys, skin, lungs, skeletal muscle, intestinal, and heart tissue) when controlled to creatures. There have all the earmarks of being immaterial entrance into the CNS. Gliclazide likewise crosses the placental obstruction and courses in the fetal blood circulation system. A low evident volume of diffusion is most likely reflected in the high level of gliclazide official to proteins (around 94% at a plasma concentration of 8mcg/mL).

2.2.8.3 Metabolism

Quickly and very much ingested yet may have wide between and approximately 70% of the administrated dosage is discharged gradually in the urine, encompassing a spike 7 to 10 hours after administration. Metabolites are perceptible in the urine 120 hours after organization. Fecal end represents roughly 11 % of the administrated dosage [5]. Gliclazide is generally totally dispensed with inside 144 hours post – dosage.

2.2.8.4 Excretion and Elimination

Metabolites and conjugates are wiped out essentially by the kidneys (60-70%) and furthermore in the dung (10-20%). The pharmacokinetics parameters of gliclazide are mentioned and shown in Table 2.

Sr. No.	Pharmacokinetics Parameter	Values
1.	Oral absorption	100%
2.	Iean elimination half-life	10.4 hours. Duration of action is 10-24 hours.
3.	Minimum effective concentration	2.2 to 8.0 µg/ml
4.	Maximum effective concentration	8.0 to 13 µg/ml
5.	Plasma protein binding	94%, highly bound to plasma proteins.

Table 2 Pharmacokinetics parameters of gliclazide.

2.2.9 Uses & Indications

Diabetes mellitus (type- II) which cannot be controlled by diet alone in the adult at the beginning stage of the disease.

2.2.10 Drug Interaction

Numerous drug interactions have been found using gliclazide by which of the curation of T2DM and their side effects can be investigate some drug interactions of this drug are mentioned in Table 3 [7].

Drug	Interaction
Acebutolol	It may decrease symptoms of hypoglycemia and increase the time required for the body to compensate for hypoglycemia.
Acetylsalicylic acid	Acetylsalicylic acid increases the effect of the sulfonylurea, gliclazide.
Atenolol	The beta-blocker, atenolol, may decrease symptoms of hypoglycemia.
Betaxolol	The beta-blocker, betaxolol, may decrease symptoms of hypoglycemia.
Bevantolol	The beta-blocker, bevantolol, may decrease symptoms of hypoglycemia.
Bismuth Subsalicylate	The salicylate, bismuth subsalicylate, increases the effect of the sulfonylurea, gliclazide.
Bisoprolol	The beta-bloker, bisoprolol, may decrease symptoms of hypoglycemia.
Carteolol	The beta-blocker, carteolol, may decrease symptoms of hypoglycemia.
Carvedilol	The beta-blocker, carvedilol, may decrease symptoms of hypoglycemia.

| Chloramphenicol | Chloramphenicol may increase the effect of sulfonylurea, gliclazide. |
| Clofibrate | Clofibrate may increase the effect of sulfonylurea, gliclazide. |

Table 3 Drug interactions of gliclazide [7].

2.2.11 Dosage and administration

The medicine dosage should be originated level at 40mg (half tablet) regularly and maybe enhance the dosage if required up to 320mg regularly (4 tablets). The dosage up to 160mg/ day may be occupied in a single day, if possible, it can be taking the same time every morning, this dosage (160mg/day) can be taken in two separated as morning and evening. The brutality of glycemia will regulate the dosage, needing modification to gain the ideal response at the minimum dosage. The usage of gliclazide does not prevent the necessity of modifying diet.

2.2.12 Toxicity

LD_{50} =3000 mg/kg (orally in mice). Gliclazide and its metabolites may collect in those with extreme hepatic or potentially renal brokenness. Side effects of hypoglycemia include dazedness, absence of vitality, sleepiness, cerebral pain, and perspiring [6].

2.2.13 Warnings and precautions

Some intense entanglements, (for example, extreme injury, fever, contamination, or medical procedure) can happen because of metabolic stress. This highlights the inclination of hyperglycemia and ketosis. Insulin must be regulated to control these circumstances. An increment in measurements of gliclazide isn't suitable. Close perception of patients through all phases of the organization, especially in old, incapacitated, malnourished, semi-starved, or the individuals who have dismissed dietary limitations, is important to guarantee that hypoglycemia doesn't happen.

2.2.14 Side effects

Major and minor side effects of gliclazide are as mentioned in Table 4.

Severe	Rare
Dizziness	Confusion
	Weakness

Nausea or vomiting	Sweating
	Changes in vision
Diarrhea	Decreased heartbeat
	Abdominal pain
	Constipation
	Skin rash
	Elevated liver enzymes

Table 4 Side effects of gliclazide.

2.2.15 Storage

The storage of this drug is to be at the room temperature in the range between 15 - 30 °C. Also keep this drug away from heat, light and dampness. Try not to store in the restroom. Keep this apart from the kids.

2.3   Glipizide

Glipizide is one of the most consistency prescribed medication for the treatment of type -II diabetes mellitus [7]. Its standard features are spready and short action with an extraordinary high selectivity [8, 9]. It is hundred times more serious than tolbutamide in moving pancreatic discharge of insulin [10]. The critical effect of glipizide is to expand insulin availability following meals, while it has little impact on evening glucose control [11]. It is used for patients with type- II diabetes who have declined diet and exercise treatment and it radiates an impression of being insulin secretagogue both; in the first stage insulin excretion and in proceeded stimulatory response during long stretch administration [12].

2.4.   Specifications of glipizide drug [13]

2.4.1   Drug Class

Blood-glucose-lowering drug of the sulfonylurea class.

2.4.2   IUPAC Name

1-Cyclohexyl-3-[[p-[2-(5-methylpyrazinecarboxamido) ethyl] phenyl] sulfonyl] urea.

2.4.3   Generic name

Glucotrol

2.4.4 Chemical formula

$C_{21}H_{27}N_5O_4S$.

2.4.5 Appearance

Opaque, Odorless powder

2.4.6 Structure Formula:

The structure of glipizide is shown in Fig. 3.

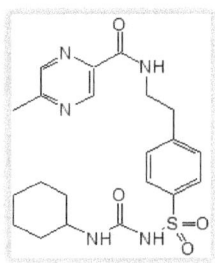

Fig. 3 Structure of glipizide drug.

2.4.7 CAS registry no

29094-61-9

2.4.8 Solubility

The solubilization of glipizide in some organic and inorganic solvents are shown and mentioned in Table 5. **[14-16]**.

Solvent Used	Solubility
Water & alcohol	Unsolvable
Acetone and Dichloromethane (DCM)	Very Slightly Soluble
Alkali Hydroxide solutions and DMF	Promptly Soluble
hloromethane and Methylene Chloride	Freely Soluble

Table 5 Solubilization data of glipizide [14-16].

2.4.9 Molecular weight

445.54 gm./mol

2.4.10 Dissociation constant (pKa)

It is a weak acid so value of pKa is 5.9 [17].

2.4. 11 Melting point

The melting point is 208- 209°C and practically reported is 200- 203°C. [18].

2.4.12 Therapeutic categories

Glipizide is under categorized to an Oral antidiabetic agent.

2.4.13 Boiling point

Not applicable

2.4.14 Mechanism action

Glipizide brings down the blood glucose by summoning the delivery of insulin from the pancreatic β-cells [19]. Like different sulphonylureas, which combine with receptors on pancreatic β-cells and block adenosine triphosphate delicate potassium channels.   This thusly prompts opening voltage delicate calcium channels which produce a deluge of calcium ions, calcium calmodulin conceiving, kinase activation and delivery of insulin containing granules by exocytosis [20,21].

2.4.15 Clinical pharmacokinetics profile of glipizide

Pharmacokinetic characteristics viz. absorption, distribution, metabolism and elimination of glipizide are summarized here.

2.4.15.1 Absorption

Glipizide is quickly and totally consumed following oral organization in a prompt discharge measurement structure. The supreme bioavailability of Glipizide was 100% after single oral portions in patients with type- II diabetes. plasma tranquilize focuses bit by bit rises arriving at greatest fixations inside 6 to 12 hours subsequent to dosing.

2.4.15.2 Distribution

Glipizide is quickly appropriated and has a little evident volume of distribution [22], bout 0.14-liter/kg with a scope of 0.07-0.19 liter/kg. Protein restricting was concentrated in serum from volunteers who got either oral or intravenous glipizide and saw as 98-99 % one hour after either course of administration **[23]**. Glipizide primarily ties to egg whites' proteins.

2.4.15.3 Metabolism

The digestion of glipizide is broad and happens basically in the liver; the liver processes the medication fundamentally into hydroxylated and conjugated subordinates, its two metabolic results are trans-4-hydroxyglipizide and cis-3-hydroxyglipizide; neither metabolite gives off an impression of being dynamic **[15,9]**. The significant metabolites of glipizide are results of sweet-smelling hydroxylation and have no hypoglycemic action. A secondary metabolite, by which represents less than 2 % of a portion, an acetylamino-ethyl benzene subordinate, is accounted for to have 1/10 to 1/3 as much hypoglycemic action as the origin compound **[24]**.

2.4.15.4 Excretion and elimination

Glipizide is wipe out principally by hepatic biotransformation, below 10% of a dose is exudate as uninterrupted medicine in urine and defecation; roughly 90% of dose is exudate as biotransformation items in urine (80%) and drug (10%) **[11]**. The half- existence of end ranges from 2- 4 hours in ordinary subjects, regardless of whether given intravenously or orally **[24]**.

However, in beginning examinations, half-existence of medication was accounted for to be 1.71-2.1 h **[25]**. The metabolic and excretory examples are comparable with the two courses of organization, showing that first pass digestion isn't significant **[22]**. Studies on renal disabled patients give data that renal deficiency doesn't influence the digestion of medication, just leeway of metabolites from blood is affected **[26]**. Different pharmacokinetic properties of glipizide are abridged in Table 6.

Sr. No.	Pharmacokinetics Parameter	Values
1.	**Oral absorption**	100%
2.	**Mean elimination half-life**	2 -4hr
3.	**ᵖre-systemic metabolism**	0%
4.	**Minimum effective concentration**	20 nm/mL

5.	**Maximum**	300 nm/mL
	effective concentration	
6.	**Plasma protein binding**	98-99%

Table 6 Pharmacokinetics properties of glipizide.

2.4.16 Uses & indications

Glipizide is indicated as an adjunct to diet and exercise to improve glycemic control in adults with type -II diabetes mellitus.

2.4.17 Dosage and administration

The most extreme suggested dosage is 40mg every day in an isolated dosage. The dosage ought to be decreased intolerance with hepatic impedance. The suggested beginning dosage is 5 mg/day up to 15 mg/day given as a solitary day by day dosage. For greatest impact in decreasing postprandial hyperglycemia, this specialist ought to be ingested 30 min before breakfast, since fast retention is postponed when the medication is taken with nourishment [27-29].

2.4.18 Drug interaction

Numerous drug interactions have been found using glipizide by which of the curation of T2DM and their side effects can be investigate some drug interactions of this drug are mentioned in Table 7 [30].

Drug	Interaction
Acebutolol	Acebutolol may decrease symptoms of hypoglycemia and increase the time required for the body to compensate for hypoglycemia.
Acetylsalicylic acid	Acetylsalicylic acid increases the effect of the sulfonylurea, Glipizide.
Atenolol	The beta-blocker, atenolol, may decrease symptoms of hypoglycemia.
Bisoprolol	The beta-blocker, bisoprolol, may decrease symptoms of hypoglycemia.

Carvedilol	The beta-blocker, carvedilol, may decrease symptoms of hypoglycemia.
Chloramphenicol	Chloramphenicol may increase the effect of sulfonylurea, Glipizide.
Clofibrate	Clofibrate may increase the effect of sulfonylurea, Glipizide.
Cyclosporine	The sulfonylurea, Glipizide, may increase the effect of cyclosporine.
Esmolol	The beta-blocker, esmolol, may decrease symptoms of hypoglycemia.
Labetalol	The beta-blocker, labetalol, may decrease symptoms of hypoglycemia.
Nadolol	The beta-blocker, nadolol, may decrease symptoms of hypoglycemia.

Table 7 Drug interactions of glipizide [30].

2.4. 19 Toxicity

Manifestations of an overdose in sulfonylureas, including glipizide, might be identified with serious hypoglycemia and may incorporate unconsciousness, seizure, or other neurological disability. These are side effects of extreme hypoglycemia and require quick treatment with glucagon or intravenous glucose and close checking for at least 24 to 48 hours since hypoglycemia may repeat after obvious clinical recuperation. Mellow hypoglycemic indications without loss of awareness or neurologic discoveries ought to be treated with oral glucose.

2.4.20 Warnings and precautions

Hepatic and renal diseases monitor blood and urinary glucose periodically.

2.4.21 Side effects

Major and minor side effects of glipizide are mentioned in Table 8.

Severe	Rare

Yellowing of skin and eyes	Diarrhea
Dark colored urine	Dizziness
	Shaking of body
Pain in upper abdomen	Skin Rash
Unusual bleeding	Excessive air or gas in stomach
Fever	Elevated liver enzymes
Decreased heartbeat	

Table 8 Side effects of glipizide.

2.4.22 Storage

Try not to store above 25°c.and keep away from sunlight.

2.5 Glimepiride

Glimepiride belongs sulfonylurea class drug of 2nd generation which is generally used in the treatment of type II diabetes mellitus. It has a place with class-II of Biopharmaceutical order framework and slightly soluble in various buffers and organic solvent [31].

2.5.1 Specifications of glimepiride

2.5.2 IUPAC name

4-ethyl-3-methyl-N-[2-[4-[(4-methylcyclohexyl) carbamoylsulfamoyl] phenyl] ethyl]-5-oxo-2H-pyrrole-1-carboxamide.

2.5.3 Generic name

Amaryl

2.5.4 Chemical formula

The chemical formula of glimepiride is $C_{24}H_{34}N_4O_5S$ [32].

2.5.5 Structure formula

The structure of glimepiride shown in Fig. 4 [33].

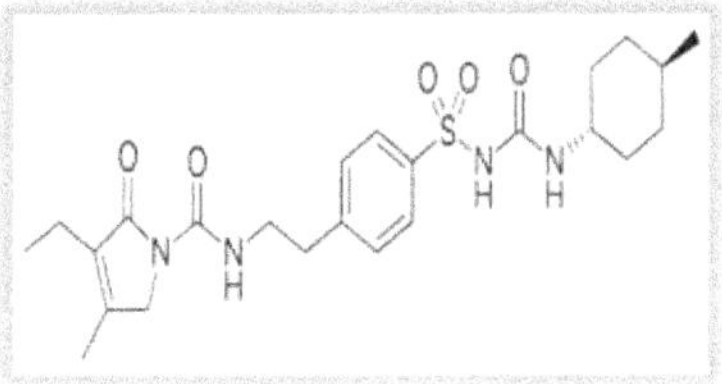

Fig. 4 Structure of glimepiride [33].

2.5.6 Appearance

Its appearance is like White to yellowish-white crystalline powder, odorless, to practically odorless powder.

2.5.7 CAS registry no

93479-97-1

2.5.8 Solubility

The solubilization of glimepiride in some organic and inorganic solvents are shown and mentioned in Table 09 [34, 35]. It shows low pH subordinate dissolvability in acidic and impartial watery media, it displays poor solvency at 37 °C (<0.004 mg/ml). In media pH>7, the dissolvability of medication is marginally expanded up to 0.002mg/ml.

Solvent Used	Solubility
Water, Acid, Base	Insoluble
Methanol, Ethanol and Acetone	Partially soluble
DMF	Fully soluble
DMSO	Fully soluble

Table 9 Solubilization data of glimepiride [34,35].

2.5.9 Spectral analysis

Methanolic solution of glimepiride drug gives UV absorptions at 229nm and the aqueous solutions of glimepiride gives λ max maximum absorption in between 229 and 236nm.

2.5.10 Therapeutic categories

Glimepiride under categorized to an Oral antidiabetic agent.

2.5.11 Dissociation constant (pKa)

14.12

2.5.12 Melting point

207°C

2.5.13 Boiling point

Not applicable

2.5.14 Mechanism action

The essential instrument of activity of Glimepiride in sinking blood glucose has all the earmarks of being subject to animate the arrival of insulin from working pancreatic beta cells. Moreover, extra-pancreatic impacts may likewise assume a job in the movement of sulfonylureas, for example, Glimepiride. This is upheld by both preclinical and clinical investigations showing that Glimepiride organization can prompt expanded affectability of fringe tissues to insulin. These discoveries are steady with the aftereffects of a long haul, randomized, fake treatment controlled preliminary in which Glimepiride treatment improved postprandial insulin/C-peptide reactions and by and large glycemic control without delivering clinically important increments in fasting insulin/C-peptide levels. Be that as it may, similarly as with different sulfonylureas, the component by which Glimepiride brings down blood glucose during long haul organization has not been unmistakably settled [36-38].

2.5. 15 Clinical pharmacokinetics profile of glimepiride

2.5.15.1 Absorption

After oral organization, Glimepiride is totally (100%) ingested from the GI tract. Studies with single oral portions in typical subjects and with different oral dosages in patients with type-II has demonstrated huge retention of Glimepiride with 1 hour after organization and pinnacle medicate levels at 2 to 3 hours [9-11].

2.5.15.2 Distribution

After intravenous (IV) dosing in ordinary subjects, the volume of dispersion (VD) was 8.8L (113ml/kg), and the complete body freedom (Cl) was 47.8 ml/min. Protein restricting was more prominent than 99.5% [9-11].

2.5.15.3 Metabolism

Glimepiride is totally utilized by oxidative bioconversion after either an IV or oral portion. The significant metabolites are the cyclohexyl hydroxyl methyl subordinate (M1) and the carboxyl subsidiary (M2). Cytochrome P450 2C9 has been established to be engaged with the bioconversion of Glimepiride to M1. M1 is additionally used to M2 by one or a few cytosolic catalysts. M1, however not M2, has around 1/3 of the pharmacological action as contrasted with its parent in a creature model [9-11].

2.5.15.4 Excretion and elimination

At the point when ^{14}C-Glimepiride was given orally, around 60% of the complete radioactivity was recuperated in the pee in 7 days and M1 (dominating) and M2 represented 80 – 90% of that recuperated in the pee. Roughly 40% of that recuperated in defecation. No parent sedate was recouped from pee or dung. The primary metabolites are inactive hydroxylation products and polar conjugates and are excreted mainly in the urine [9-11].

2.5.16 Uses & indications

Glimepiride is shown as an aide to eat fewer carbs and exercise to bring down the blood glucose in persistent with type-II diabetes mellitus. Hypoglycemia can't be constrained by diet and exercise alone. Glimepiride might be utilized correspondingly with Metformin when starve, exercise, Glimepiride or Metformin alone don't satisfactory glycemic control [9-11].

2.5.17 Drug interaction

Numerous drug interactions have been found using glimepiride by which of the curation of T2DM and their side effects can be investigate some drug interactions of this drug are mentioned in Table 10.

Drug	Interaction
Cyclosporine	The sulfonylurea, glimepiride may increase the effect of cyclosporine.
Gemfibrozil	Gemfibrozil increases the effect and toxicity of pioglitazone/ rosiglitazone
Glucosamine	Possible hyperglycemia
Ketoconazole	Ketoconazole increases the effect of rosiglitazone
Rifampin	Rifampin may decrease the effect of sulfonylurea, glimepiride.

Somatropin recombinant	Somatropin may antagonize the hypoglycemic effect of glimepiride. Monitor for changes in fasting and postprandial blood sugars

Table 10 Drug interaction of glimepiride.

2.5.18 Dosage and administration

The regular beginning portion of Glimepiride's introductory treatment is 1mg to 2mg once day by day, controlled with breakfast or first primary feast. Quiet who might be progressively touchy to hypoglycemic medications ought to be begun at1mg once day by day, and ought to be titrated cautiously. The most extreme beginning portion of Glimepiride ought not to be more than 2mg. The common upkeep portion is 1 to 4mg once day by day. The most extreme suggested portion is 8mg once every day.

2.5.19 Toxicity

Side impacts from taking glimepiride incorporate gastrointestinal tract (GI unsettling influence, and once in a while thrombocytopenia, leukopenia, hemolytic sickliness, and sometimes unfavorably susceptible responses happen. In the underlying long stretches of treatment, the danger of hypoglycemia might be expanded. Liquor utilization and introduction to daylight ought to be limited in patients taking it since they can intensify the symptoms.

2.5.20 Side effects

Major & minor side effects for glimepiride are mentioned in Table 11.

Severe	Rare
Hypoglycemia,	Dizziness
Elevated liver enzymes,	Headache
Anemia,	Nausea
Jaundice	Asthenia
	Flu like symptoms
	Allergic skin reaction

| Weight gain |

Table 11 Side effects of glimepiride.

2.5.21 Storage

Storage of this drug at room temperature around 25 – 30 °C, also father from direct light and dampness, keep farther from kids.

2.6. Glibenclamide (AKA Glyburide)

Glibenclamide is an oral antihyperglycemic operator utilized for the curation of non-insulin-subordinate diabetes mellitus (NIDDM).

2.6.1 Specifications of glibenclamide

2.6.2 Class

Generation-II Sulfonylurea Antidiabetics.

2.6.3 IUPAC name

5-chloro-N-[2-(4-{[(cyclohexylcarbamoyl)amino]ulfonyl}phenyl)ethyl]-2-methoxybenzamide

2.6.4 Generic name

Glyburide

2.6.5 Chemical formula

$C_{23}H_{28}ClN_3O_5S$

2.6.6 CAS registry no

10238-21-8

2.6.7 Molecular weight

494.041gm/mol

2.6.8 Chemical structure

Chemical structure of glibenclamide are shown in Fig.5 **[39].**

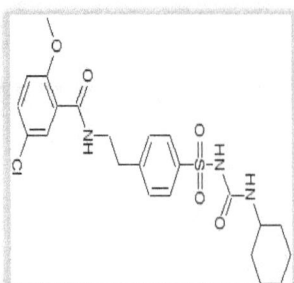

Fig. 5 Structure of glibenclamide [39].

2.6.9 Physicochemical properties of glibenclamide

2.6.10 Appearance

A white or almost white, crystalline powder.

2.6.11 Melting point

169 °C

2.6.12 Solubility

The solubilization of glimepiride in some organic and inorganic solvents are shown and mentioned in Table 12.

Solvent Used	Solubility
Water & alcohol	Insoluble
Methylene chloride	Freely soluble
Methanol	Slightly soluble

Table 12 Solubilization data of glibenclamide.

2.6.13 Dissociation Constatnt (pKa)

4.32

2.6.14 Storage

Try not to store above 25°c.and keep away from sunlight.

2.6.15 Therapeutic categories

Glibenclamide is under categorized to an Oral antidiabetic agent.

2.6.16 Boiling point

Not applicable

2.6.17 Mechanism of action

Sulfonylureas comparatively as Glibenclamide tie to ATP- delicate potassium channels on the pancreatic cell surface, diminishing potassium conductance and causing depolarization of the film(membrane). Depolarization animates calcium particle ion influx through voltage- delicate calcium channels, raising intracellular conc. of calcium particles, which prompts the emission or exocytosis of insulin.

2.6.18 Clinical pharmacokinetics properties of glibenclamide

2.6.18.1 Absorption

Gastrointestinal retention is uniform, fast, and basically complete.

2.6.18.2 Distribution

After ingestion sedate bound to plasma protein and reach to the site of activity.

2.6.18.3 Metabolism

Basically hepatic (Frequently cytochrome P450 3A4). The significant metabolite is the 4-trans-hydroxy subordinate. A subsequent metabolite, the 3-cis-hydroxy subsidiary, likewise happens. These metabolites don't contribute clinically critical hypoglycemic activity in people as they are just pitifully dynamic; be that as it may, maintenance of 4-trans-hydroxyglyburide may draw out the hypoglycemic impact of the operator in those with serious renal impedance.

2.6.18.4 Excretion and elimination

Glyburide is discharged as metabolites in the bile and pee, around half by each course. This double excretory pathway is subjectively not quite the same as that of different sulfonylureas, which are discharged essentially in the urine. The pharmacokinetics parameters for the glibenclamide are mentioned in Table 13.

Sr. No.	Pharmacokinetics Parameter	Values
1.	Oral absorption	100%
2.	Mean elimination half-life	1.4 to 1.8 hours.
3.	Plasma	99%, highly bound

| protein binding | to plasma proteins. |

Table 13 Pharmacokinetics parameters of glibenclamide.

2.6.19 Uses & indications

Shown as an assistant to eat fewer carbs to bring down the blood glucose in patients with NIDDM whose hyperglycemia can't be acceptably constrained by diet alone.

2.6.20 Drug interactions

Numerous drug interactions have been found using glibenclamide by which of the curation of T2DM and their side effects can be investigate some drug interactions of this drug are mentioned in Table 14 **[39]**.

Drugs	Interaction
Acebutolol	Acebutolol may decrease symptoms of hypoglycemia and increase the time required for the body to compensate for hypoglycemia.
Acetylsalicylic Acid	Acetylsalicylic acid increases the effect of the sulfonylurea, glibenclamide.
Atenolol	The beta-blocker, atenolol, may decrease symptoms of hypoglycemia.
Betaxolol	The beta-blocker, betaxolol, may decrease symptoms of hypoglycemia.
Bevantolol	The beta-blocker, bevantolol, may decrease symptoms of hypoglycemia.
Bismuth Subsalicylate	The salicylate, bismuth subsalicylate, increases the effect of the sulfonylurea, glibenclamide.
Bisoprolol	The beta-blocker, bisoprolol, may decrease symptoms of hypoglycemia.
Bosentan	Increased risk of hepatic toxicity

Table 14 Drug interaction of glibenclamide.

2.6.21 Dosage and administration

The prescribed beginning dosage is 2.5 to 5 mg day by day of customary tablets or 1.5-3 mg every day of micronized tablets. The most extreme dosage is 1.25 to 20 mg of normal tablets and 0.75 to 12 mg of micronized tablets. Glibenclamide normally is directed with the principal primary feast of the day.

2.6.22 Toxicity

The oral LD_{50} in rodents is >3200mg/kg, in mice is >1500mg/kg, in hares is >10,000mg/kg, and in guinea pigs is >1500mg/kg [40]. Patients encountering an overdose may give hypoglycemia [41]. Mild hypoglycemia ought to be treated with oral glucose and changes in accordance with medicating dosages or supper schedules [41]. Severe hypoglycemia may give trance-like state, seizure, and neurological impairment [41]. This ought to be dealt with promptly in an emergency clinic with intravenous glucose and observing for 24-48 hours.

2.6.23 Warning and precautions

To accomplish the objective of treatment with Glibenclamide ideal control of blood glucose - adherence to right eating regimen, standard and adequate physical exercise and, if essential, decrease of body weight are similarly as important as normal ingestion of Glibenclamide.

2.6.24 Side effects

Major and minor side effects of glibenclamide are mentioned in Table 15.

Severe	Rare
Yellowing of skin and eyes	Nausea
Dark colored urine	Heartburn
Fever or chills	Abdominal fullness
Swelling of face, lips,	Fast heartbeat
eyelids, tongue, hands and feet	Unusual tiredness and weakness
Unusual bleeding	

Table 15 Side effects of glibenclamide.

2.6.25 Storage

Customary or Micronized Tablets All around shut compartments at 15–30°C. Fixed-mix Tablets Light-safe compartments up to 25°C.

3. CONCLUSION

With conclusion, I have expansively overviewed the antidiabetic medicines used for the curation of diabetes type-II mellitus. This overview provides the crucial information the above-mentioned drugs of glimepiride, gliclazide, glipizide, and glibenclamide availability, their pharmacokinetics and pharmacodynamics properties, clinical properties, that causes side effects.

4. DECLARATION OF INTEREST

None

5. ACKNOWLEDGEMENT

The authors are thankful to the V.P & R.P.T.P science college for providing the research facilities and also very thankful to the management C.V.M., Vallabh Vidhyanagar.

6. REFERENCES

1. Pizzi RA. Defying diabetes: The discovery of insulin. Mod. Drug Discovery.2000; (3): 77-80.

2. Leahy JL, Cooper HE, Deal DA, Weir GC. Chronic hyperglycemia is associated with impaired glucose influence on insulin secretion. A study in normal rats using chronic in vivo glucose infusions. J Clin Invest 1986 ;77(3):908-15.

3. Bell GI, Polonsky KS. Diabetes mellitus and genetically programmed defects in β-cell function. Nature 2001;414(6865):788-91.

4. Baba S. Double-blind randomized control study with gliclazide Clin Eva 1983; 11(1):51-94.

5. Ings RMJ, Campbell B, Gordon BH, Beaufils M, Meyrier A, Jones R: The effect of renal disease on the pharmacokinetics of gliclazide in diabetic patients Br J Clin Pharmacol 1986; 21(5):572-573.

6. Jerums G, Murray RM, Seeman E, Cooper ME, Edgley S, Marwick K, Larkins RG, Martin TJ. Lack of effect of gliclazide on early diabetic nephropathy and retinopathy: a two-year controlled study. Diabetes Res Clin Pract 1987;3(2):71-80.

7. https://www.drugbank.ca/drugs/DB01120

8. H. O. Ammar, H. A. Salama, M. Ghorab, S. A. El-Nahhas and H. Elmotasem. Curr Drug Deliv 2006; 3(3):333.

9. Colin Dollery. Therapeutic Drugs, 2nd Ed., Churchill Livingstone; 1999;(1):56.

10. Prabhu P, Harish NM, Gulzar AM, Yadav B, Narayana CR, Satyanarayana D, Subrahmanayam EV. Formulation and in vitro evaluation of gastric oral floating tablets of glipizide. Indian J Pharm Educ Res 2008;42(2):174-183.

11. Semalty M, Semalty A, Kumar G. Formulation and characterization of mucoadhesive buccal films of glipizide. Indian J Pharm Sci 2008;70(1):43-58

12. Wåhlin-Boll E, Groop L, Karhumaa S, Groop PH, Tötterman KJ, Melander A. Therapeutic equivalence of once-and thrice-daily glipizide. Eur J Clin Pharmacol 1986;31(1):95-99.

13. Sankalia JM, Sankalia MG, Mashru RC. Drug release and swelling kinetics of directly compressed glipizide sustained-release matrices: Establishment of level A IVIVC. J Control Release 2008;129(1):49-58.

14. Remington: "The Science and Practice of Pharmacy" Mack Publishing Company, Pennsylvania; 18042, Vol-II, chap-2 1080-1081 p.

15. Pfizer. Glucotrol XLR Glipizide Extended Release Tablets Prescribing Information, New York, NY, May (2007).

16. Sean C. Sweetman, Martindale, The Complete Drug Reference, 35th Ed. Pharmaceutical Press, London, (2007) p. 400.

17. Kaynak MS, Kaş HS, Öner L. Formulation of controlled release glipizide pellets using pan coating method. Hacettepe University Journal of the Faculty of Pharmacy 2007;27(2):93-106.

18. Shivakumar, H. N., Patel, P. B., Desai, B. G., Ashok, P. and Arulmozhi, S. Design and statistical optimization of glipizide loaded lipospheres using response surface methodlogy. Acta Pharm 2007; 57: 269-285.

19. The Merck Index, 13th Ed., Merck and Co Inc. Whitehouse Station 790, NJ, USA. (2001).

20. David R. Williams and Thomas L. Lemke, Foye's Principles of Medicinal Chemistry, 5th Ed., Lippincott William and Wilkins, (2005) p. 629.

21. Thomson Micromedex, Drug Information for Health Care Professional, 24th Ed., Vol I, (2004) p. 296.

22. Merck Sante Metaglip™ (Glipizide and Metformin HCl) Tablets Prescribing Information Darmstadt, Germany (2002).

23. Wåhlin-Boll E, Almér LO, Melander A. Bioavailability, pharmacokinetics and effects of glipizide in type 2 diabetics. Clin pharmacokinet 1982;7(4):363-372.

24. Brogden RN, Heel RC, Pakes GE, Speight TM, Avery GS. Glipizide: a review of its pharmacological properties and therapeutic use. Drugs 1979;18(5):329-353.

25. Ambrogi V, Bloch K, Daturi S, Logemann W, Parenti MA. Synthesis of pyrazine derivatives as potential hypoglycemic agents. J Pharm Sci 1972;61(9):1483-1486.

26. Balant L, Zahnd G, Gorgia A, Schwarz R, Fabre J. Pharmacokinetics of glipizide in man: influence of renal insufficiency. Diabetologia 1973;9(1):331-338.

27. Antidiabetics, in Martindale "The Extra Pharmacopoeia" 1999. Royal Pharmaceutical Society, 32nd Edition, 320p.

28. Hardman J G, limbird L.E. Godman and Gilman's "The Pharmacological Basis of Therapeutics" 10th Edition. New York; Me Graw Hill; 2001.

29. Tripathi K D, "Essential of medical pharmacology" 4th Edition, New Delhi, Jaypee Brothers (p) Ltd; 1994.

30. https://www.drugbank.ca/drugs/DB01067

31. Kishore K, Sudhakara RP, Srininvas RD, Maneshwar T, Kiran KV, Raju L, Preparation and characterization of oro dispersible tablets of glimepiride- pvp k30 solid dispersion, Int J Bio Pharm Res 2013; 4(8): 547-555.

32. Chowdary KP, Vijayasrinivas S. Biopharmaceutical classification system. The Indian Pharmacist 2004;3(30):7-10.

33. https://www.drugbank.ca/drugs/DB00222

34. Saroj B, Mahesh KK, Ajay B. An overview on solid dispersion techniques implemented for dissolution enhancement of glimepiride. Am J Pharmatech Res 2014; 4: 65-77.

35. Rani GS, Lohita M, Preethi PJ, Madhavi R, Sunisitha B, Mounika D. Glimepiride: a review of analytical methods. Asian J Pharm Anal 2014;4(4):178-182.

36. British Pharmacopoeia Commission. British Pharmacopoeia, vol. 1. London: 2003. p. 874–875.

37. United States of Pharmacopoeia, (2004). Asian edition. 866-867,1922.

38. AHFS Drug Information, (2004). 3033-3040, 2567-2569.

39. https://www.drugbank.ca/drugs/DB010166

40. https://pfe-pfizercom-d8-prod.s3.amazonaws.com/products/material_safety_data/MICRONASE.pdf

41. https://www.accessdata.fda.gov/drugsatfda_docs/label/2009/017532s030lbl.pdf

Publisher: Eliva Press SRL

Email: info@elivapress.com

Eliva Press is an independent publishing house established for the publication and dissemination of academic works all over the world. Company provides high quality and professional service for all of our authors.

Our Services:
Free of charge, open-minded, eco-friendly, innovational.

-Free standard publishing services (manuscript review, step-by-step book preparation, publication, distribution, and marketing).
-No financial risk. The author is not obliged to pay any hidden fees for publication.
-Editors. Dedicated editors will assist step by step through the projects.
-Money paid to the author for every book sold. Up to 50% royalties guaranteed.
-ISBN (International Standard Book Number). We assign a unique ISBN to every Eliva Press book.
-Digital archive storage. Books will be available online for a long time. We don't need to have a stock of our titles. No unsold copies. Eliva Press uses environment friendly print on demand technology that limits the needs of publishing business. We care about environment and share these principles with our customers.
-Cover design. Cover art is designed by a professional designer.
-Worldwide distribution. We continue expanding our distribution channels to make sure that all readers have access to our books.

www.elivapress.com